INTRODUCTIN

Saxenda (liraglutide) is used for weight loss and to help maintain weight off once weight has been misplaced, it is used for overweight adults or overweight adults who additionally have weight-related medical problems. Saxenda can be used in youngsters aged 12 to 17 years who with weight problems and who've a bodyweight above 132 pounds (60 kg). Saxenda is used together with a healthful food regimen and exercise. Saxenda is an injection given as soon as a day below the skin (subcutaneous) from a multi-dose injection pen.

Saxenda includes the same lively ingredient (liraglutide) as Victoza. The difference among Saxenda and Victoza is they are exceptional strengths and they may be FDA authorized for different conditions. Saxenda is not for treating kind 1 or kind 2 diabetes. It isn't always regarded if Saxenda is safe and powerful in youngsters less than 12 years of age. It isn't always recognized if Saxenda is secure and powerful in youngsters elderly 12 to 17 years with kind 2 diabetes.

BEFORE THE USAGE OF SAXENDA

You have to not use Saxenda if you are allergic to liraglutide, or if you have:

• More than one endocrine neoplasia kind 2 (tumors on your glands);

• A non-public or family history of medullary thyroid carcinoma (a type of thyroid cancer); or

• Diabetic ketoacidosis (call your health practitioner for remedy). You need to now not use Saxenda if you also use insulin or different drug treatments like liraglutide (albiglutide, dulaglutide, exenatide, Byetta, Bydureon, Tanzeum, Trulicity).

To make sure Saxenda is safe for you, inform your health practitioner if you have:

- belly problems inflicting slow digestion;

- Kidney or liver disorder;

- High triglycerides (a type of fat in the blood);

- Coronary heart problems;

- A records of troubles together with your pancreas or gallbladder; or

- A history of despair or suicidal thoughts. In animal research, liraglutide caused thyroid tumors or thyroid cancer. It is not acknowledged whether or not these results would arise in people the use of normal doses. Ask your doctor about your risk. It isn't always regarded whether Saxenda will damage an unborn child. Tell your physician if you are pregnant or plan to come to be pregnant. It isn't regarded whether liraglutide passes into breast milk or if it could have an effect on the nursing baby. Tell your doctor in case you are breast-feeding.

Saxenda isn't always FDA-approved for use through everybody more youthful than 18 years old.

Saxenda is commonly given once according to day. Follow all instructions for your prescription label. Your medical doctor may now and again alternate your dose. Do not use this remedy in large or smaller amounts or for longer than encouraged. Do not use Saxenda and Victoza together. These two brands incorporate the equal active factor however they have to not be used together. Read all affected person information, medication publications, and practise sheets supplied to you. Ask your doctor or pharmacist if you have any questions. Saxenda is injected below the skin at any time of the day, without or with a meal. You will be proven how to use injections at home. Do no longer self-inject this medicine if you do not understand how to deliver the injection and nicely remove used needles and syringes. Saxenda comes in a prefilled injection pen. Ask your pharmacist which type of needles is best to apply along with your pen. Your card issuer will show you the pleasant locations to your body to inject Saxenda. Use an exceptional area whenever you supply an injection. Do no longer inject into the identical location two instances in a row. Do no longer use Saxenda if it has changed colors or if it has particles in it. Call your pharmacist for new medication. Also look ahead to symptoms of excessive blood sugar (hyperglycemia) inclusive of elevated thirst or urination, blurred imaginative and prescient, headache, and tiredness. Blood sugar ranges can be laid low with pressure, illness, surgical operation, workout, alcohol use, or skipping food. Ask your doctor before converting your dose or medication time table. Use a disposable needle simplest once.

Follow any state or neighborhood legal guidelines approximately throwing away used needles and syringes. Use a puncture-proof "sharps" disposal container (ask your pharmacist where to get one and the way to throw it away). Keep this container out of the attain of children and pets. Saxenda is best part of a entire treatment application which could additionally include weight loss program, exercise, weight manage, normal blood sugar testing, and unique hospital therapy. Follow your health practitioner's commands very intently.

Storing unopened injection pens: Store inside the fridge. Do not freeze Saxenda, and throw away the medicine if it has turn out to be frozen. Do not use an unopened injection pen if the expiration date at the label has handed. Storing after your first use: You may keep "in-use" injection pens in the refrigerator or at room temperature. Protect the pens from moisture, warmth, and daylight. Use within 30 days. Remove the needle earlier than storing an injection pen, and maintain the cap on the pen when not in use.

SAXENDA FACET EFFECTS

Get emergency medical assist if you have symptoms of an hypersensitive reaction to Saxenda: hives; speedy heartbeats; dizziness; hassle respiration or swallowing; swelling of your face, lips, tongue, or throat.

Call your medical doctor straight away if you have:

• racing or pounding heartbeats;

• Surprising modifications in mood or behavior, suicidal thoughts;

- Excessive ongoing nausea, vomiting, or diarrhea;

- Signs and symptoms of a thyroid tumor - swelling or a lump to your neck, trouble swallowing, a hoarse voice, feeling quick of breathe;

- Gallbladder troubles - fever, top belly ache, clay-colored stools, jaundice (yellowing of your pores and skin or eyes);

- symptoms of pancreatitis - extreme ache on your higher stomach spreading to your lower back, nausea without or with vomiting, fast coronary heart charge;

- critically low blood sugar - intense weak spot, confusion, tremors, sweating, rapid heart rate, hassle talking, nausea, vomiting, fast respiratory, fainting, and seizure (convulsions); or

- Kidney problems - little or no urination; painful or hard urination; swelling in your toes or ankles; feeling tired or brief of breath. Common Saxenda facet outcomes might also encompass:

- Nausea (specially while you begin the use of Saxenda), vomiting, belly pain;

- multiplied heart price;

- Diarrhea, constipation;

- Headache, dizziness; or

- Feeling tired.

This isn't always an entire list of facet outcomes and others may additionally occur. Call your doctor for medical advice about aspect outcomes. You may also report aspect results to FDA at 1-800-FDA-1088.

WHAT OTHER TABLETS WILL HAVE AN EFFECT ON SAXENDA?

Saxenda can slow your digestion, and it can take longer in your frame to soak up any medicines you take by using mouth. Tell your doctor approximately all of your current medicines and any you start or stop using, in particular:

- Insulin; or

- Oral diabetes medicine - Glucotrol, Metaglip, Amaryl, Avandaryl, Duetact, DiaBeta, Micronase, Glucovance, and others.

This listing isn't always whole. Other capsules may additionally interact with liraglutide, together with prescription and over the counter medicines, nutrients, and natural merchandise. Not all viable interactions are indexed in this medication guide.

WHO IS SAXENDA RECOMMENDED FOR?

Saxenda is FDA-approved for use inside the following individuals primarily based on frame mass index (BMI):

• Adults with overweight (BMI of 27 or greater) and at the least one weight-related condition (inclusive of high blood pressure of type 2 diabetes)

• Adults with weight problems (BMI of 30 or more)

• Adolescents 12 to 17 years old with obesity Pediatric obesity is described as a BMI inside the 95th percentile or extra for age and sex, says Dr. Mann. The manufacturer labeling additionally consists of a minimum pediatric weight requirement above 132 pounds. Saxenda is not encouraged for individuals with a private or own family records of medullary thyroid most cancers, says Dr. Mann, and in people with a rare, hereditary endocrine disorder called a couple of endocrine neoplasia (MEN 2). "It is also contraindicated in being pregnant," she says. According to the producer (Novo Nordisk), Saxenda additionally hasn't been studied for use for the duration of lactation.

Always seek advice from your health practitioner approximately any concerns you can have earlier than beginning a new medicinal drug.

WHAT IS THAT THIS MEDICINE?

LIRAGLUTIDE (LIR a GLOO tide) promotes weight loss. It may also be used to hold weight loss. It works by using lowering urge for food. Changes to diet and workout are regularly mixed with this medicine. This remedy can be used for other functions; ask your fitness care provider or pharmacist if you have questions.

COMMON BRAND NAME(S): Saxenda

WHAT NEED TO I INFORM MY CARE GROUP EARLIER THAN I TAKE THIS MEDICATION?

They want to know if you have any of those situations:

- Endocrine tumors (MEN 2) or if a person for your circle of relatives had those tumors

- Gallbladder disorder

- High cholesterol

- History of alcohol abuse hassle

- History of pancreatitis

- Kidney ailment or in case you are on dialysis

- Liver ailment

- Previous swelling of the tongue, face, or lips with issue respiration, trouble swallowing, hoarseness, or tightening of the throat

- Stomach troubles

- Suicidal mind, plans, or attempt; a preceding suicide try by way of you or a member of the family

- Thyroid most cancers or if someone for your circle of relatives had thyroid most cancers

- An uncommon or allergy to liraglutide, other medicines, foods, dyes, or preservatives

- Pregnant or trying to get pregnant

- Breast-feeding

HOW MUST I USE THIS MEDICINAL DRUG?

This medication is for injection below the pores and skin of your upper leg, stomach location, or higher arm. You will be taught how to put together and give this medicinal drug. Use precisely as directed. Take your medicinal drug at everyday intervals. Do no longer take it greater frequently than directed. This medication comes with INSTRUCTIONS FOR USE. Ask your pharmacist for directions on the way to use this medicinal drug. Read the information carefully. Talk to your pharmacist or care team when you have questions. It is vital which you put your used needles and syringes in a unique sharps container. Do now not position them in a trash can. If you do no longer have a sharps container, name your pharmacist or care crew to get one. A unique Med Guide can be given to you by the pharmacist with every prescription and top off. Be certain to read this information cautiously on every occasion. Talk on your care crew about the use of this medicine in youngsters. While it may be prescribed for children as young as 12 years of age for selected conditions, precautions do apply.

Overdosage: If you watched you've got taken an excessive amount of of this medicine touch a poison manage middle or emergency room right now. NOTE: This medication is most effective for you. Do now not proportion this medicinal drug with others.

WHAT HAVE TO I LOOK AHEAD TO WHILE THE USAGE OF THIS MEDICINAL DRUG?

Visit your care group for regular checks in your development. Drink lots of fluids whilst taking this remedy. Check with your care crew if you get an attack of severe diarrhea, nausea, and vomiting. The lack of too much body fluid can make it dangerous if you want to take this medicinal drug. This medicine may additionally have an effect on blood sugar stages. Ask your care crew if modifications in diet or medications are needed if you have diabetes.

Patients and their families should watch out for worsening depression or thoughts of suicide. Also watch out for surprising modifications in emotions consisting of feeling tense, agitated, panicky, irritable, antagonistic, aggressive, impulsive, critically restless, overly excited and hyperactive, or now not being capable of sleep. If this takes place, especially at the start of remedy or after a trade in dose, name your care group. Women must inform their care team in the event that they wish to come to be pregnant or think they is probably pregnant. Losing weight while pregnant isn't always recommended and might reason harm to the unborn infant. Talk to your care team for greater records.

WHAT FACET CONSEQUENCES MAY ALSO I WORD FROM RECEIVING THIS MEDICINAL DRUG?

Side results which you should file to your care team as soon as viable:

- Allergic reactions or angioedema—skin rash, itching, hives, swelling of the face, eyes, lips, tongue, palms, or legs, trouble swallowing or breathing

- Fast or irregular heartbeat

- Gallbladder issues—severe belly ache, nausea, vomiting, fever

- Kidney harm—lower in the quantity of urine, swelling of the ankles, palms, or feet

- Pancreatitis—severe belly ache that spreads to your lower back or receives worse after eating or whilst touched, fever, nausea, vomiting

- Thoughts of suicide or self-harm, worsening mood, emotions of depression

- Thyroid most cancers—new mass or lump within the neck, pain or trouble swallowing, problem breathing, hoarseness

Side results that typically do now not require scientific attention (report on your care group in the event that they retain or are bothersome):

- Constipation

- Dizziness

- Fatigue

- Headache

- Loss of Appetite

- Nausea

- Upset stomach

This list may not describe all feasible facet outcomes. Call your health practitioner for medical recommendation about facet consequences. You may also document side consequences to FDA at 1-800-FDA-1088.

WHERE OUGHT TO I MAINTAIN MY REMEDY?

Keep out of the attain of youngsters and pets. Store unopened pen in a refrigerator among 2 and 8 stages C (36 and 46 levels F). Do not freeze or use if the drugs has been frozen. Protect from light and immoderate heat. After you first use the pen, it may be saved at room temperature between 15 and 30 ranges C (fifty nine and 86 levels F) or in a fridge. Throw away your used pen after 30 days or after the expiration date, whichever comes first. Do now not shop your pen with the needle connected. If the needle is left on, medication might also leak from the pen. NOTE: This sheet is a summary. It won't cover all possible information. If you've got questions about this medicine, communicate for your medical doctor, pharmacist, or health care provider.

WHAT MAY ADDITIONALLY INTERACT WITH THIS MEDICATION?

• Insulin and different medicines for diabetes

This listing might not describe all viable interactions. Give your fitness care issuer a list of all the medicines, herbs, non-pharmaceuticals, or nutritional dietary supplements you operate. Also tell them if you smoke, drink alcohol, or use illegal drugs. Some items may also have interaction along with your medicine.

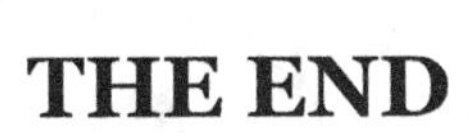
THE END